SYMPTOMS AND SIGNS OF
SUBSTANCE MISUSE

2nd Edition

SYMPTOMS AND SIGNS OF SUBSTANCE MISUSE

2nd Edition

Dr Margaret M. Stark LLM DGM DMJ DAB
Honorary Senior Lecturer
The Forensic Medicine Unit
St George's Hospital Medical School, London, UK
stark@cheam.demon.co.uk

Dr J. Jason Payne-James LLM FRCS DFM RNutr
Forensic Physician, London
Forensic Medical Examiner, Metropolitan Police
Service & City of London Police
Director, Forensic Healthcare Services Ltd
jasonpaynejames@aol.com

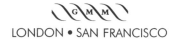
LONDON • SAN FRANCISCO

© 2003

Greenwich Medical Media Limited

137 Euston Road
London
NW1 2AA

870 Market Street, Ste 720
San Francisco, CA 94102

ISBN 1841101060

First Edition Published 1996
Second Edition Published 2003

Typeset by Mizpah Publishing Services, Chennai, India
Printed in the UK by The Cromwell Press
Distributed by Plymbridge Distributors and in the USA by JAMCO Distribution
Visit our website at **www.greenwich-medical.co.uk**

CONTENTS

INTRODUCTION

There are few parts of society in most countries of the world that are not touched by some aspect of substance misuse. The misuse of both illicit and licit drugs is widespread. The term substance misuse is a general term to describe the misuse of drugs. Drugs (those legally prescribed and illegally supplied) including alcohol and tobacco all have the potential for being misused. Individuals may use drugs occasionally (so-called 'recreational' use) may become addicted to or dependent upon certain drugs. Drugs may affect home, school, work, sporting and personal life. Dependence or addiction may be physical, psychological or both. The undesirable and unwanted effects differ from drug to drug – individuals may describe physical or psychological effects that they feel or experience – 'symptoms', or others may see or observe physical effects – 'signs'. The widespread availability and enormous variety of drugs – many used in combination – with many different effects can make it difficult to recognize if drugs are being used, or, if a drug is being used, what type it is. This small book is intended to provide concise and readily accessible facts about the symptoms and signs associated with the most commonly misused drug groups to assist healthcare professionals, employers, police, parents, teachers, partners, or friends in identifying whether drugs are being misused. The range and mix of drugs means that few signs and symptoms are diagnostic, and if drugs are suspected further specialist help should be sought from those experienced in the management of substance misuse. The book also summarises the different types of drugs, how they produce their effect, and methods of treatment or management.

The issues are also placed into the context of current law in England and Wales. The medical and clinical principles are similar throughout the world.

For those wishing to explore some of these issues further, a reading list of suitable texts for more detailed or specialised information is given on page 50.

METHODS OF ADMINISTRATION

Drugs – licit or illicit – may be taken or administered in a number of ways. The main routes are: orally – by mouth (sometimes placed under the tongue – 'sublingually'), intra (or per-)nasally – inhaled as a pure drug into the nose ('sniffed', 'snorted'); or by burning the drug and inhaling the fumes ('chasing', 'chasing the dragon'); smoking – by mixing the drug with tobacco in a cigarette and inhaling the smoke; intravenously – by injecting a liquid form or solution of the drug into a vein ('mainlining', 'fixing'), subcutaneously ('skinpopping') – injecting into the tissue just below the skin or intramuscular – injecting through skin and subcutaneous tissues into the muscle. In a small proportion of cases, vaginal and rectal administration – placement of the drug directly into the vagina or rectum – is used and in these cases the drug may be absorbed rapidly across the mucosal lining. Some drugs (e.g. cocaine powder) may be applied directly to the gums to achieve a very rapid effect. An increasingly common problem is that of swallowing drugs in packages, either in an attempt to conceal drugs ('swallowers', or to smuggle drugs ('stuffers', 'mules', 'body packers'), and leakage of the contents of such packages – even in small quantities can be fatal. If swallowing or stuffing is suspected – immediate medical advice should be sought from a unit with full resuscitation facilities. Drugs may be concealed in any body orifice including, mouth, ears, vagina, rectum, nose and beneath the foreskin. Drugs have also been concealed in stomas.

HARM MINIMISATION AND REDUCTION

For many individuals misusing drugs the choice of total avoidance of the drug is not possible. It is unrealistic to believe that substance misuse will not occur. It is now recognised that for those individuals who will continue to use drugs it is desirable to try and reduce the amount of harm that may ensue to both the individual and the community. This approach has been termed either harm minimisation or harm reduction.

Examples of harm to the individual include the development of hepatitis or HIV infection secondary to the sharing of non-sterile needles and syringes to inject drugs. An example of harm to the community includes the accidental needle-stick injury sustained as a result of discarded injection materials left in public places. A number of initiatives have been used to combat specific areas of potential harm. The provision of needle and syringe exchange centres in the community is one such initiative.

The use of hepatitis B immunisation programmes for intravenous drug misusers, reduces the risk of infection to the individual, and may benefit the community by reducing costs by avoiding the need for long-term hospital care.

Awareness of harm minimisation methods are important for the drug misuser, their healthcare team, friends and family.

Other health promotion strategies should be considered when assessing any suspected substance misuser including offering treatment or advising on other medical problems; referral to local agencies/drug arrest referral schemes; advice can be given on injecting practices including the avoidance of 'shared works'; education on the risk of overdose including loss of tolerance and multiple drug use; increase the general awareness of blood-borne viruses and sexual health issues including contraception and sexually transmitted diseases.

DRUGS, STATUTES AND LEGAL REQUIREMENTS

This section refers to the laws of England and Wales. Readers outside this jurisdiction should acquaint themselves with local laws relating to drugs and drug use. Drugs (both prescribed and non-prescribed) are subject to certain legal controls. Import and export of drugs controlled under these Acts is within the jurisdiction of Her Majesty's (HM) Customs and Excise under the Customs & Excise Management Act 1979.

PRESCRIBING CONTROLLED DRUGS

A Home Office licence is required to prescribe heroin, cocaine, dipipanone or any of their salts to a person addicted to these drugs (although they can be prescribed for organic disease or injury). When prescribing controlled drugs certain regulations apply. The prescription should be in ink and hand written with the address of the prescriber, signed and dated. The name and address of the patient stating the drug, the form, strength (where appropriate), dose, number of dosage units or the total quantity given in words and figures must be supplied.

MISUSE OF DRUGS ACT 1971

The Act provides the legal framework for the control of drugs and details the specific requirements for the prescription, safe custody, record-keeping and the offences relating to production, cultivation, supply and possession of most drugs. Penalties for contravention of sections of the Misuse of Drugs statutes and regulations can be severe ranging up to life imprisonment for supplying (selling or giving away) a Class A drug (see Table 1).

Table 1 Misuse of Drugs Act 1971

Penalty purposes	
Class A	major natural and synthetic opiates (specified by name)
	cocaine
	lysergic acid diethylamide (LSD)
	injectable amphetamines
	cannabinol and derivatives
	methylenedioxymethamphetamine (MDMA)
Class B	oral amphetamines
	cannabis plant material and resin
	codeine, dihydrocodeine
	methylphenobarbitone, pentazocine
Class C	benzodiazepines, anabolic steroids
	buprenorphine, dextropropoxyphene
	cathinone

MISUSE OF DRUGS REGULATIONS 1985

These regulations provide schedules which define certain classes of persons who may possess, produce, supply, prescribe or administer certain drugs in the practice of their professions (see Table 2).

MEDICINES ACT 1968

The Medicines Act 1968 lays down how medicines are produced and supplied. Medicines are divided into three categories under the Act.

- General Sales List (GSL) – medicines which can be sold from any premises without supervision or advice from a doctor or pharmacist.
- Pharmacy Medicines (PM) – can only be obtained from a pharmacy and are sold under the supervision of a pharmacist.
- Prescription Only Medicines (POM) – must be prescribed by a doctor, a dentist or, in exceptional circumstances, another health professional.

HEALTH AND SAFETY AT WORK ACT 1974

The Health and Safety at Work Act 1974 places responsibilities on both employers to ensure the health, safety and welfare of the employees as far as is reasonably practical, and employees have a responsibility to take care of their own safety and fellow employees. Clearly the use of drugs or alcohol by employees or knowledge by the employer of such use could mean that either or both are not fulfilling their duties under the Act. There is increasing recognition of this fact and pre-employment screening or

Table 2 Misuse of Drugs Regulations 1985

Control purposes

Schedule 1	Prohibited drugs except with Home Office authority, e.g. cannabis, LSD, raw opium, ecstasy
Schedule 2	Full Controlled Drug requirements in relation to prescribing, safe custody, keeping of registers, e.g. diamorphine, pethidine, cocaine, amphetamine
Schedule 3	Barbiturates, meprobamate, pentazocine, temazepam and flunitrazepam
Schedule 4	Benzodiazepines (except temazepam and flunitrazepam), anabolic steroids
Schedule 5	Preparations containing small amounts of controlled drugs

workplace testing programmes are becoming more common, or actual conditions of employment.

ROAD TRAFFIC ACT 1988

Section 5(1)(a) of the Road Traffic Act 1988 states that a person commits an offence if he drives or attempts to drive a motor vehicle on a road or other public place when his alcohol level exceeds the limits prescribed below:

35 µg of alcohol in 100 ml of breath
80 mg per 100 ml of blood
107 mg per 100 ml of urine.

Section 4(1) of the Road Traffic Act 1988, as amended by s4 of the Road Traffic Act 1991 states that a person commits an offence if he drives or attempts to drive a mechanically propelled vehicle on a road or other public place when unfit through drink or drugs.

Section 4(2) of the Road Traffic Act as amended by s4 of the Road Traffic Act 1991 states that a person commits an offence if he is in charge of a mechanically propelled vehicle on a road or other public place when unfit through drink or drugs.

The extent of driving under the influence of drugs, either prescribed or illicit, and often combinations of substances, is difficult to quantify. Certain police officers are trained to identify drivers who may be impaired through drugs using Drug Recognition Training (DRT) and Field Impairment Testing (FIT) systems. See also page 54.

TRANSPORT AND WORKS ACT 1992

Section 27(1) of the Transport and Works Act 1992 states that it is an offence for any of the following persons to carry out their work while unfit through drink or drugs, namely a train or tram driver, guard, conductor or signalman or anybody who works on a transport system in which he can control or affect the movement of a vehicle or works in a maintenance capacity or as a supervisor or lookout for persons working in a maintenance capacity.

Under Section 27(2) of the same Act it is an offence for these persons to carry out their work after having consumed more alcohol than the prescribed limit.

INTOXICATING SUBSTANCES [SUPPLY] ACT 1985

This Act applies to England and Wales, and makes it an offence for a person to supply or to offer to supply to someone under the age of 18 substances which are not controlled drugs if the supplier knows or has reason to believe that the substance or the fumes from that substance will be used to achieve intoxication.

SOLVENT ABUSE (SCOTLAND) ACT 1983

The Solvent Abuse (Scotland) Act 1983 made solvent sniffing one of the grounds for referring a young person to a Children's Panel via the Reporter. This Panel is a semi-judicial body to whom children who commit certain offences or who are otherwise felt to be in need of care may be referred.

MEDICAL AND HEALTH COMPLICATIONS OF SUBSTANCE MISUSE

Substance misuse can result in medical and other health complications that may be specific to the particular substance of misuse, or may be generic – in that they are caused by the mode of substance misuse. Such complications may be the first indicator of a substance misuse problem in the absence of acute or chronic symptoms and signs of specific drugs.

Any known or suspected drug misuser should have a full history taken and clinical examination at regular intervals to determine the risks or establish the presence of any treatable or new complication. The history should ascertain what drugs are being used, by what route, how frequently, how much, how recently and whether other drugs are being used concurrently (both prescribed and illicit – not omitting alcohol and tobacco). The physical examination should also establish whether there is clinical evidence of whether the individual is intoxicated or withdrawing from a drug at that time. The physical examination should look at all parts of the body – as stigmata of drug misuse such as needle marks and needle tracks may be concealed. If there is clear evidence of current intoxication it is appropriate to document baseline conscious level, using the Glasgow Coma Score (see page 53) (although it is important to be aware that the Score is specifically for head injury and not validated for those under the influence of drugs or alcohol).

Habitual smokers of certain drugs develop chronic wheezy chests, which may be improved by abstinence from the drug, or from bronchodilators. Many individuals who have smoked or chased heroin or crack cocaine can have intermittently wheezy chests (the former more pronounced during withdrawal).

Many drugs can be injected – many of the injection-related complications, irrespective of the drug injected, are caused by either sharing, or repeated use of non-sterile needles (see Harm Minimisation and Reduction). Particulate contaminants of drugs injected are also a major cause of complications – such contaminants include those that are used to mix or dilute the drug prior to street sale – and include substances such as washing powder or talcum powder. Table 3 lists the most common medical complications of drug misuse and some of the rarer conditions that should be looked for at assessment.

Table 3 Potential medical complications of drug misuse

Vascular
May be short-term, or long-term:
- accidental intra-arterial (as opposed to intravenous) injection may cause vascular spasm with ischaemia
- false aneurysm
- thrombophlebitis
- thrombosis
- embolus

Vascular spasm, thrombosis and embolus if severe and untreated can result in gangrene and loss of digits or limbs.

Intravenous injection may be followed by:
- localised superficial thrombophlebitis
- deep vein thrombosis
- pulmonary embolism

Chronic complications include:
- limb swelling (a mixture of lymphoedema and post-phlebitic changes)
- varicose eczema
- varicose ulcers

Infective complications of injection

Short-term complications:
- abscess
- bacteraemia/septicaemia
- cellulitis (local – chemical and infective)
- thrombophlebitis

MEDICAL AND HEALTH COMPLICATIONS OF SUBSTANCE MISUSE *continued*

Table 3 *continued*

Long-term complications:

- endocarditis (always look for splinter haemorrhages, anaemia)
- hepatitis
  - A (several large outbreaks have occurred in intravenous drug users (IVDUs))
  - B (10–15% in IVDUs)
  - C (up to 80% in IVDUs)
  - chronic hepatitis – chronic persistent hepatitis (relatively benign) and chronic active hepatitis (progressive), cirrhosis and primary hepatocellular carcinoma may result
  - delta virus infection may be superimposed on hepatitis B infection
- deep injection causing primary or haematogenous septicaemia
- human immunodeficiency virus (HIV) (1% overall. 3.5% in London; previously up to 90% of users in Edinburgh and Dundee were infected in the 1980s – most have now died)
- necrotising fasciitis
- osteomyelitis (haematogenous)
- respiratory
  - lung abscess
  - tuberculosis (associated with poor living conditions, malnutrition and immunological suppression)
  - septic arthritis

Non-infective complications

- anaphylaxis
- constipation (chronic opiate use)
- dental decay (especially with methadone use)
- local tissue ulceration (at injection site)
- malnutrition
- overdose (accidental)
- pneumothorax (after forced inhalation of drugs such as cocaine)
- pulmonary infarction
- respiratory wheeze (non-infective – worse on withdrawal from opiates)

SUBSTANCE DETECTION

Differentiation must be made between the qualitative and quantitative detection of drugs. Qualitative tests will solely detect the presence or absence of a drug. Some tests set a level below which the result is reported as negative. It is thus important to understand the method and means of assay and reporting, which may vary from laboratory to laboratory. This may have relevance when attempting to determine whether a drug has been used, to assist in the healthcare and medical management of an individual, or to assist control of drug misuse by occupational health teams, general practitioners, drug clinics, employers, police, schools and family. There are ethical, moral and statutory issues that must be considered. The human rights and civil liberties of the individual should be protected, but equally others who might be affected by an individual's drug misuse need to be protected, explaining the increasing use of pre-employment, on-site and random screening for drugs. Qualitative drug assays may be required for research, disciplinary, analytical and statutory purposes.

Drug detection assays are undertaken using standard methods including thin layer, high performance and gas liquid chromatography. Other methods available include techniques such as radioimmunoassay, enzyme immunoassay, fluorescence immunoassay and mass spectrometry.

Urine, saliva, blood or hair can be used for drug detection and the results can give some indications of the type, amount and time at which certain drugs were taken. In general opioids and stimulants are detectable in plasma and saliva for up to 12 h after ingestion, and in urine for days or perhaps weeks (for some drugs e.g. cannabinoids). Hair may be used to assess drug usage for up to a year. Each of these analyses require expert interpretation as the relevance of drug levels is dependent on a wide range of factors including the drug pharmacokinetics (see Table 4). Increasingly sophisticated but simple-to-use devices can be used for the immediate testing of urine for specific drugs or their metabolites, and also for the testing of surfaces such as skin, clothes, furniture or personal effects.

When substance misuse is suspected a sample of blood and urine should be taken (unless the incident was more than 4 days prior to the examination when only urine is required). In view of the short half-life of some substances the urine specimen should be taken as soon as practically possible, an approach that is particularly useful when investigating drug-facilitated sexual assault.

Table 4 Peak effect, half-life, duration of action and times for detection of common drugs

Drug	Peak effect (min)	Half-life (h)	Duration (h)	Detection possible
Cannabis	10–30	4	2–3	Up to 12 days in blood Up to 46 days in urine
Dihydrocodeine	90–120	3–4.5	3–6	12 h in blood
Methadone	60–300	12–18 after single dose 15–60 after multiple doses	36–48	48 h in blood and urine
Morphine	60	3	3–6	18 h in blood 2 days in urine
Diamorphine	30 after oral dose	3 min	3–6	40 h in urine
Diazepam	30–120	20–50	4–8	48 h in blood 1–2 days in urine
Temazepam	45–300	13	4–8	48 h in blood 1–2 days in urine
Ecstasy	120	7	4–6	48 h in blood 2–4 days in urine
Amphetamine	variable	12	2–4	48 h in blood 2–4 days in urine
LSD	30–480	2–5	3–12	2–3 days in urine
Cocaine				
– snort	30–40	1	1–1.5	12 h in blood
– intravenous	10–20			12 h–3 days in urine

(note the above figures are approximate and may vary from individual to individual).

Adapted from: A Physician's Guide to Clinical Forensic Medicine, Stark MM (ed), Human Press, Totowa, New Jersey, 2000.

SUMMARY OF INFORMATION ON EACH DRUG GROUP

The following pages give summaries of each drug and drug group. It must be emphasised that the signs and symptoms of substance misuse described refer to the use of that drug alone. Many users of drugs do not use one drug at a time. The effects noted in any given individual may relate to mixed drug use and this must always be considered when the signs and symptoms appear to be confused or contradictory.

DETAILS OF INFORMATION ON EACH DRUG GROUP INCLUDE (WHERE RELEVANT)

Principal drugs and derivatives
Manufacture
Common street names (these vary depending on region – and change
   frequently – the most common and well-established are given)
Mechanism of action (if known)
Medical uses (if any)
Legal status (in England and Wales)
Presentation and methods of administration
Symptoms and signs
   – acute intoxication
   – chronic use
   – withdrawal
Management
   – intoxication
   – general
   – chronic use
   – withdrawal

DRUG GROUP

ALCOHOL

Principal drugs

Ethyl alcohol (ethanol), methyl alcohol.

Common street names
Booze, sauce (dependent on type of alcohol).

Mechanism of action
Central nervous system (CNS) depressant potentiating gamma-aminobutyric acid (GABA) activity. Apparent stimulant effect caused by depression of inhibition (cortical) centres. It is absorbed into the blood stream and starts to have an effect within 5–10 min. The blood alcohol level peaks within 30–60 min (range 20 min–3 h) after drinking. The rate of absorption is affected by many factors including gender, weight, duration of drinking, nature of drink consumed, consumption of food, physiological factors, genetic variation, other drugs and rate of elimination. Rate of elimination is 10–25 mg/100 ml blood per hour (average ~15 mg/100 ml/h = ~1 unit/h in a 70 kg male) and is dependent on some of the above factors and related to the individual's drinking habits. A regular drinker will metabolise alcohol more quickly: 5–10% excreted unchanged in breath, urine and sweat; 90–95% oxidised in liver (enzyme = alcohol dehydrogenase) to form acetaldehyde – further metabolised to acetate. Fatal dose in adults ~6–10 ml/kg body weight.

Medical uses
There are no recommended medical uses.

Legal status
The manufacture, sale and purchase of alcoholic beverages are controlled by various licensing regulations. The substance can be bought by adults over 18 years. Offences exist such as being drunk in a public place, drunk in charge of a child under 7 years of age, drunk and disorderly, drunk and incapable or driving whilst unfit to do so because of drink (or drugs).

Presentation and methods of administration
Liquid taken orally. Concentration of alcohol in drink varies – average examples – spirits 40%, sherry 20%, wine 11–13% and beer 3–8%. One unit of alcohol contains 8 g of pure spirit and is approximately equivalent to one half a pint of beer, a single measure of spirits (e.g. brandy, whisky, gin), a small glass of sherry or a glass of wine. In Europe alcohol is labeled

according to percentage of alcohol by volume (ml pure alcohol/100ml of drink).

Symptoms and signs

Acute intoxication
- Physical: dysarthria, reddened conjunctivae, sluggish pupillary response to light, pupils normal size or dilated, nystagmus ('positional alcohol' – secondary to direct effect on vestibular system – and 'horizontal gaze' secondary to inhibition of smooth pursuit and effect on neural control of ocular movement), loss of co-ordination and ataxia, rapid full-bounding pulse, small increase in blood pressure, possible hypoglycaemia (secondary to gluconeogenesis inhibition).
- Psychological: stimulatory effects as a result of disinhibition of the higher brain centres, relief of tension and anxiety, relaxation, aggression may occur.

If alcohol is taken with other depressant drugs (in particular barbiturates) or other sedatives, such as benzodiazepines, opioids, anti-histamines or solvents, there is an increase in the depressant effects on the CNS (medullary) with greater risk of significant intoxication and overdose with cardiac and respiratory depression.

Chronic
- Signs associated with chronic misuse (but not necessarily alcohol-induced) include: plethoric facies, telangiectasia and spider naevi, reddened conjunctivae, smell of stale alcoholic liquor, acne rosacea, palmar erythema, Dupuytren's contracture, obesity, gynaecomastia, striae, bruising/scars from recurrent falls (X-ray may reveal old fractures – particularly ribs).
- Medical complications associated directly or indirectly with long-term excessive alcohol include: oesophagitis, gastritis, pancreatitis, alcoholic hepatitis and cirrhosis, dementia, encephalopathy, peripheral neuropathy and myopathy, subdural haematoma, hypertension, cardiomyopathy, cardiac dysrhythmias, tuberculosis, gout, osteoporosis, carcinoma of oropharynx, oesophagus and liver.

Tolerance to alcohol develops with repeated doses and there is a strong physical dependence.

ALCOHOL *continued*

Withdrawal

- Uncomplicated alcohol withdrawal usually occurs after 24 h with nausea, vomiting, malaise, weakness, autonomic hyperactivity (hypertension, tachycardia, sweating, anxiety), depressed mood, irritability, transient hallucinations and illusions, headache and insomnia.
- Delirium tremens ('DT's) starts 72–96 h after the last alcohol ingestion with profound disorientation and confusion with hallucinations (of any sensory modality), dilated pupils, fever, tachycardia and hypertension. Mortality of 5%. Hospitalisation required.

Other complications include convulsions, Wernicke's encephalopathy, Korsakoff's psychosis, alcoholic hallucinosis and cardiac dysrhythmias.

Treatment

General

- Simple intoxication usually requires no treatment.
- For comatose patients, general management of respiratory depression and cardiovascular collapse may be required. Treatment of hypoglycaemia may be required.
- Consideration should be given to the administration of Vitamin B as soon as possible.

Withdrawal and rehabilitation

- Detoxification should be with a long-acting benzodiazepine such as chlordiazepoxide or diazepam.
- There are a number of alcohol deterrent drugs (e.g. disulfiram, citrated calcium carbimide) which act by inhibition of aldehyde dehydrogenase. Inhibition caused by disulfiram takes several days to elapse. Very unpleasant symptoms occur after a small amount of alcohol such as flushing, headache, palpitations, nausea and vomiting and with larger doses dysrhythmias, hypertension and collapse. An information card should be carried warning of the dangers of administration of alcohol.
- Further relapse may be prevented by counselling, more intensive psychotherapy or self-help organisations such as Alcoholics Anonymous. Often such interventions require repeated and reinforced intervention. Brief interventions have been found to be useful.

Screening tests such as AUDIT, CAGE or Brief MAST may help identify those with alcohol dependency as opposed to alcohol misuse.

AMPHETAMINES

Principal drugs and derivatives

Amphetamine, methamphetamine, dexamphetamine sulphate (Dexedrine™), methylphenidate (Ritalin™).

Manufacture
Laboratory based (legal and illegal).

Common street names
Uppers, 'A', speed, wake-up, cranks, whizz, sulph, hearts, dex/dexy/dexies (Dexedrine™), crystal/ice/glass/meth (methamphetamine).

Mechanism of action
CNS stimulants (actions resemble those of adrenaline) similar to cocaine but the half-life and duration of euphoric effects are both longer. The effect is immediate by injection; oral within 30 min and when sniffed within 20 min. The effects last 4–6 h.

Medical uses
Some are indicated for the treatment of narcolepsy and is also indicated for children with refractory hyperkinetic states under the supervision of a physician specialising in child psychiatry.

Legal status
POM controlled under the Misuse of Drugs Act 1971, Class B under Schedule 2 (amphetamine, methamphetamine, dextroamphetamine, methylphenidate). All are Class A if prepared for injection.

Presentation and methods of administration
Tablets, capsules, powder, crystal 'ice' (methamphetamine hydrochloride very pure form). Also seen as a 'putty like substance' – base. May be taken orally, sniffed, snorted, smoked or injected. Street amphetamine seized by the police has a purity of about 5% (in the UK in the year 2000) compared to Customs seizures of 13% illustrating the extent to which certain drugs are cut prior to distribution by the dealers.

Symptoms and signs

Acute intoxication – effects similar to cocaine
- Physical: dry mouth, loss of appetite, sweating, dilated pupils, tachycardia, increased blood pressure. Higher doses cardiac dysrhythmias, seizures and excited delirium; rarely cerebral vasculitis and intracranial haemorrhage.

AMPHETAMINES *continued*

- Psychological: euphoria, feeling of self-confidence, raised self-esteem, lowered anxiety, increased energy, greater concentration, irritability, restlessness. Higher doses can result in irrational behaviour, confusion, fear, hallucinations, delusions, paranoia, psychosis.

Tolerance occurs with long-term use as does psychological dependence.

When injected the user additionally experiences a sensory 'rush' or 'flash' – giving almost immediate sensations of enhanced energy and self-confidence. The 'high' reported with smoking methylamphetamine is supposedly more intense than cocaine.

General/chronic
- Long-term use requires increased dosage levels due to tolerance, with progression to intravenous use. 'Speed runs' describe the repeated use over a period of days. Several grams of amphetamines may be used daily. At the end of the 'run' the user may sleep for several days. Often associated with excess alcohol, use of barbiturates, benzodiazepines or heroin to reduce anxiety caused by amphetamines. Amphetamines may also be used to reduce the sedative effects of alcohol or heroin.
- Physical: long-term use may additionally cause anorexia and weight loss, malnutrition, vomiting, cardiac dysrhythmias, cardiomyopathy, angina, diarrhoea, convulsions, formication, coma and death.
- Psychological: in addition to the short-term effects continued amphetamine usage can cause aggression, fatigue, weakness, insomnia, anxiety, depression, suicidal ideation, psychosis (drug induced or trigger latent schizophrenia).

Cessation/withdrawal
- Users find that cessation can cause craving, anxiety, depression for periods of months, disturbance of sleep patterns, irritability, suicidal ideation and deliberate self-harm.

Treatment

Intoxication: nil – unless complications develop. Then supportive care with monitoring of vital signs in hospital setting. Psychosis usually resolves once the drug has been eliminated.

- General/chronic: as for intoxication.

- Withdrawal: psychological support and counselling. Insomnia and depression may require symptomatic treatment. Individuals at risk of self-harm should be carefully assessed.

ANABOLIC STEROIDS

Principal drugs

Testosterone, nandrolene, stanozolol, Durabolin™, Deca-Durabolin™.

Mechanism of action
Hormones with anabolic and androgenic effects.

Medical uses
Used in the treatment of some aplastic anaemias; osteoporosis – but no longer recommended; to reduce the itching of chronic biliary obstruction.

Legal status
POM under the Medicines Act 1968 and controlled under the Misuse of Drugs Act 1971 Class C.

Presentation and method of administration
Taken orally and can be injected. May be taken cyclically with different steroids used simultaneously – 'stacking' or use increasing doses of a given drug – 'pyramid'. They are taken by body builders and athletes to enhance their physical appearance.

Symptoms and signs

- Physical: hypertrophied muscles, hypertension, abnormal liver function tests, jaundice, peliosis hepatitis, liver tumours, Wilm's tumours, reduction of high-density lipoprotein (HDL), increase in low-density lipoprotein (LDL) cholesterol, thrombosis, reduction in testosterone resulting in a decrease in sperm quality and output, testicular atrophy, gynaecomastia, acne, striae, hirsutism, deepening of voice (higher doses), male pattern baldness and decreased breast size in women. Stigmata of injecting with usual risks of HIV, AIDS and hepatitis.
- Psychological: euphoria, anxiety, irritability, increase in aggression 'roid rage', confusion, sleep disorder, depression, psychosis.

ANABOLIC STEROIDS *continued*

Treatment

The drugs should be stopped immediately. Liver function tests usually return to normal. Withdrawal symptoms such as craving, depression and fatigue may occur.

Gynaecomastia may not resolve spontaneously and may require surgical excision for cosmetic reasons.

BARBITURATES

Principal drugs

Amylobarbitone (Amytal™); pentobarbitone (Nembutal™); quinalbarbitone (Seconal™); butobarbitone (Soneryl™); Tuinal™ contains sodium salts of amylobarbitone and quinalbarbitone.

Common street names
Downers, barbs, barbies.

Mechanism of action
Sedative-hypnotic drugs that depress the CNS potentiating the effects of the inhibitory neurotransmitter GABA.

Medical uses
The intermediate acting barbiturates should only be used for cases of severe intractable insomnia in patients already taking the drugs. The long-acting barbiturates such as phenobarbitone are used for epilepsy and rarely misused. The very short-acting drugs such as thiopentone are used for anaesthesia.

Legal status
POM controlled under the Misuse of Drugs Act 1971.

Presentation and methods of administration
Oral (pills, capsules, elixir); injection.

Less commonly encountered since the introduction of benzodiazepines; however they may be used with other drugs, in particular heroin.

Symptoms and signs

Acute intoxication
• Physical: sedation, with increasing doses: slurred speech, loss of co-ordination, ataxic gait, coma and death. There is a narrow margin

BARBITURATES *continued*

between the therapeutic and lethal doses. The risks of complications from injection are increased as these substances are poorly soluble.
- Psychological: anxiolytic, impairment of memory and cognition.

Chronic
- Sedative-hypnotic drugs cause physical and psychological dependence and an abstinence syndrome. Chronic intoxication occurs as there is an upper limit to tolerance with sedative-hypnotic drugs and individuals often increase their regular consumption above this point. There may be nystagmus, difficulty with accommodation (the ability to focus), ataxia; with higher doses – drowsiness, coma and death.
- Withdrawal starts within 24 h with anxiety, tremor, insomnia, restlessness, tachycardia; blood pressure, respiration rate and temperature may be slightly raised. Epileptiform fits may occur, especially with persistent tachycardia (>100 beats per minute).

Treatment

Cross-tolerance exists between the different barbiturates; any barbiturate can be used to treat the withdrawal syndrome of another (benzodiazepines may also be used).

If dependent on prescribed drugs, gradual reduction over several weeks or months may be possible. If large doses are used, often obtained from illicit sources, then it may be more appropriate that detoxification should be carried out within hospital.

Treatment should be aimed at preventing the medical complications of fits and psychosis with a long-acting benzodiazepine such as diazepam.

BENZODIAZEPINES

Principal drugs

Chlordiazepoxide, diazepam, clonazepam, lorazepam, temazepam, oxazepam, flunitrazepam, nitrazepam, midazolam.

Zopiclone, zaleplon and zolpidem are respectively a cyclopyrrolone, a pyrazolopyrimidine and an imidazopyridine. All are used for short-term treatment of insomnia and act on benzodiazepine receptors.

Common street names
Tranx, benzos, jellies, eggs, temazzies, mazzies, blueys, blue bomb.

BENZODIAZEPINES *continued*

Mechanism of action

These sedative-hypnotic drugs depress the CNS.

The benzodiazepines produce the pharmacological effects by enhancing GABA transmission and therefore abrupt cessation of the drugs will result in a reduction in GABA function.

Short- and medium-acting drugs include lorazepam, oxazepam and temazepam with a duration effect of 6–12 h. They are therefore taken 3 or 4 times a day.

Long-acting drugs with a half-life of over 12 h include diazepam, nitrazepam and chlordiazepoxide, usually taken once a day for sleeping.

Medical uses

The benzodiazepines are used as anxiolytic and sedative drugs. They are also useful for the treatment of muscle spasm. Some benzodiazepines such as clonazepam may be used in the treatment of epilepsy.

Diazepam and others may be used as a premedication before operations or other diagnostic procedures.

The Committee on Safety of Medicine (CSM) in the United Kingdom has issued advice on the prescribing of these drugs:

1. Benzodiazepines are indicated for the short-term relief (2–4 weeks only) of anxiety that is severe, disabling or subjecting the individual to unacceptable distress occurring alone or in association with insomnia or short-term psychosomatic, organic or psychotic illness.
2. The use of benzodiazepines to treat short-term 'mild' anxiety is inappropriate and unsuitable.
3. Benzodiazepines should be used to treat insomnia only when it is severe, disabling or subjecting the individual to extreme distress.

Legal status

POM controlled under the Misuse of Drugs Act Class C and under the Misuse of Drugs Regulations 1985 Schedule 4 (except temazepam and flunitrazepam which has recently been rescheduled into Schedule 3, making it an offence to possess the drug without a prescription).

Presentation and methods of administration

Tablets, liquid or capsules. Taken orally or injected.

Symptoms and signs

Acute intoxication
- Physical: dizziness, sedation, loss of co-ordination, dysarthria, nystagmus, confusion, impairment of skilled task performance.
- High doses (overdose) – may have low blood pressure; respiratory depression; coma; hyporeflexia. Death is unusual with benzodiazepines alone.
- Psychological: relief of anxiety, promote relaxation, memory impairment – anterograde amnesia – from the time of administration till the blood level falls.

There may be a 'paradoxical' behavioural response with increased aggression and hostility. Uncharacteristic events may occur: uncontrollable emotional responses such as giggling or weeping.

There is a 'hang-over' effect even in low dosage. The following day there may be drowsiness, inability to concentrate and impairment of tasks such as driving or operating machinery.

Alcohol and benzodiazepines increase each other's actions and marked impairment can occur. The effects of other drugs including analgesics, anti-depressants and anti-histamines, may be enhanced.

The shorter-acting benzodiazepines have been particularly implicated as potential agents for drug-facilitated sexual assault.

Chronic
- Tolerance develops rapidly to both the sedative and anxiolytic effects. Cross-tolerance exists between the benzodiazepines, alcohol and other non-barbiturate hypnotics, including chlormethiazole. Physical and psychological dependence occurs with chronic intoxication in those who regularly take large doses.
- Chronic intoxication occurs as there is an upper limit to tolerance to sedative-hypnotic drugs and dependent individuals increase their daily consumption beyond this. The clinical manifestations are not unlike alcohol intoxication with slurred speech, difficulty in concentration, poor comprehension, memory impairment, emotional lability with irritability and depressed mood.
- Withdrawal symptoms occur in 20–40% of long-term users who have received therapeutic doses for 4–6 months. Symptoms may occur within 2–3 days of stopping the short-acting drugs and within 7–10 days of stopping the longer-acting-drugs.

BENZODIAZEPINES *continued*

Table 5 Dose equivalence of benzodiazepines

	Drug	Dose
5 mg of diazepam is equivalent to:	Chlordiazepoxide	15 mg
	Loprazolam	0.5–1 mg
	Lorazepam	500 μg
	Lormetazepam	0.5–1 mg
	Nitrazepam	5 mg
	Oxazepam	15 mg
	Temazepam	10 mg

The withdrawal syndrome results in anxiety, sweating, insomnia, headache, tremor, nausea; disordered perceptions including feelings of unreality, abnormal bodily sensations, hypersensitivity to stimuli; psychosis and convulsions.

Treatment

- Intoxication: flumazenil is a specific benzodiazepine antagonist that produces rapid reversal of sedation. However it must not be used in patients with a history of fits, concurrent use of tricyclic anti-depressants, or previous toxin-induced cardiotoxicity. Should be used where resuscitation procedures are available. Re-sedation may occur after reversal, particularly when longer-acting benzodiazepines are involved.
- Withdrawal: change onto a long-acting benzodiazepine such as diazepam and reduce dose over a period of time (see Table 5 for dose equivalences). High dose dependency may require in-patient detoxification.

CANNABIS

Principal drugs

Cannabis is derived from *Cannabis sativa plant*. It refers to a range of presentations. The most important active ingredients are the tetracannabinols (THC) – particularly delta-9-tetrahydrocannabinol.

CANNABIS *continued*

Common street names
Pot, dope, blow (sometimes also used for cocaine), grass, marijuana, ganja, weed, skunk, hash, hashish (resin), draw, puff, nabis, skunk, Moroccan, Lebanese Red, Lebanese Gold.

Mechanism of action
THCs are absorbed very quickly in the lungs and the plasma concentration peaks quickly within 10–30 min, so the effects of a cigarette containing cannabis (typically 10–20 mg THC) will be felt within minutes and last for 2–3 h. If ingested the onset of action is slower, a larger dose will be needed to achieve the same effects which will then last longer. THCs and their metabolites are extremely soluble and will therefore remain for long periods of time in the fatty tissues of the body. A single dose may take 30 days for complete elimination, and chronic ingestion may lead to an accumulation of THCs and metabolites in the body.

Medical uses
There are no recommended medical uses but claims have been made that cannabis may help symptoms such as muscle spasm in patients with multiple sclerosis and for the nausea induced after chemotherapy. Clinical trials are exploring these issues.

Legal status
Cannabis is a controlled drug under the Misuse of Drugs Act 1971. It is illegal to grow, possess or supply the drug. The Home Office can grant a licence for special purposes such as research. Herbal cannabis (except seeds and stalks), cannabis resin and cannabis oil are classified as Class B drugs whereas the active chemical ingredients (cannabinoids) that have been separated from the plant are classified as Class A drugs. There are government proposals to reclassify cannabis to Class C.

Presentation and methods of administration
'Hashish' or 'hash' is a resin and is the commonest type of cannabis in the UK.

Herbal cannabis, also known as 'grass', 'dope', 'ganja', is a green coloured preparation made from the leaves of the plant.

Cannabis oil is the strongest preparation and is less common in the UK.

Cannabis is usually smoked in a cigarette (spliffs, joints, roaches) but it can be ingested in liquid form or put into food (e.g. cakes). It is the most widely misused controlled drug in the UK.

'Skunk' is derived from cannabis plants that have been selectively grown to produce a high content of THC – it is particularly potent.

CANNABIS *continued*

Symptoms and signs

Acute intoxication
- Physical: dryness of the mouth, increased appetite ('munchies'), dysarthria, ataxia, reddened conjunctivae, increased blood pressure associated with postural hypotension, tachycardia.
- Psychological: a feeling of well-being, relaxation, euphoria, increased self-confidence, perceptions of senses (e.g. smell and taste) may be altered or enhanced. There may be poor concentration, drowsiness, memory impairment, suggestibility and difficulty with tasks requiring manual dexterity. The ability to drive a car may be adversely affected. Occasionally anxiety, agitation and paranoia or a toxic psychosis may occur. Flashbacks may occur after the effects of the drugs wear off and probably when other drugs such as LSD have been used. Psychosis may occur after consumption of a large quantity of cannabis. Confusion occurs suddenly and is associated with delusions, paranoia, time and space distortion, hallucinations, emotional lability. There may be temporary amnesia with disorientation and depersonalisation. This appears to be a dose-related effect and therefore is not common in the UK where the THC content of cannabis is low when compared to that in the West Indies or India. Those with pre-existing mental illness may develop a cannabis-induced functional psychosis which responds swiftly to anti-psychotic medication but tends to relapse with resumption of cannabis usage.

Chronic
- There is no conclusive evidence that cannabis use causes physical or mental health problems in the long-term. 'Amotivational' syndrome is a rare condition where chronic apathy is attributed to long-term heavy cannabis use. Whether this condition actually exists and is related to cannabis use is controversial. Frequent inhalation of cannabis smoke over a long period may result in respiratory problems such as bronchitis and perhaps lung cancer (although this may relate in part to tobacco). High dosage chronic use may result in reduced testosterone and sperm count, reduced fertility in women, premature birth with a corresponding reduction in fetal birth weight. Gynaecomastia may occur. There may be an effect on the immune system making users more susceptible to bacterial infections. There have been suggestions that prolonged use of cannabis may lead to brain damage but there is no conclusive evidence as yet for this being the case. Long-term studies are required to explore this. Tolerance develops rapidly within a few days of regular drug use and decays rapidly when drug use ceases. With very heavy use physical

CANNABIS *continued*

dependence may occur with a mild abstinence syndrome starting a few hours after stopping the drug and lasting for four or five days.
• Withdrawal can result in irritability, restlessness, decreased appetite and weight loss.

Treatment

There is no specific treatment.

COCAINE

Cocaine is prepared from the erythroxylum coca bush and is usually found as a white odourless, bitter powder, cocaine hydrochloride.

Principal drugs and derivatives

Benzoylmethylecognine (pure), cocaine hydrochloride.

Manufacture

Refined through number of purification stages in illegal factories from leaves to paste to cocaine hydrochloride. Freebase is produced by dissolving cocaine hydrochloride in water and heating it with baking powder or ammonia to free the cocaine alkaloid base from the salt, this makes it easier to burn and therefore smoke. The name crack comes from the sound of burning sodium chloride (table salt) left when baking soda is used.

Common street names

Coke, 'C', charlie, wash, nose-candy, crack, rock, snow, stone, washed rock, base.

Mechanism of action

CNS stimulant. The onset of action, half-life and duration of effects depend on the route of administration. When sniffed, effects are felt within a few minutes and last up to half an hour, and doses may have to be repeated every 20 min. If smoked the effects are immediate and last 10–15 min.

Medical uses

As a surface anaesthetic (e.g. in ear/nose/throat surgery), may be prescribed (rarely) by doctors with a special licence from the Home Office for the treatment of addiction.

COCAINE *continued*

Legal status
POM, controlled under Class A Schedule 2 of the Misuse of Drugs Act 1971.

Presentation and methods of administration
Leaves of the coca plant which may be chewed or taken as tea (uncommon outside countries of origin in South America); as coca paste – a smokeable form used mainly where the plant grows; white crystals/powder (cocaine hydrochloride) which may be snorted through a straw or rolled up paper – in 'lines'; or from a small 'coke spoon', may be injected into veins; or applied to mucous membranes; crack may be smoked in cigarettes or pipe, may be mixed with heroin and injected ('speedballing' or 'snowballing'). Homemade pipes may be made from a variety of readily available items such as glass or plastic bottles and silver foil and even asthma inhalers.

Street cocaine seized by the police has a purity of about 52% (in the UK in the year 2000) compared to Customs seizures of 67% illustrating the extent to which certain drugs are cut prior to distribution by the dealers.

Symptoms and signs

Acute intoxication – similar to amphetamine.
- Physical: the effects are short-acting, but dose-dependent. The user may experience tachycardia, sweating, pupillary dilation, pyrexia, reduced appetite, reduced need for sleep. Higher doses lead to cardiac dysrhythmias, seizures and excited delirium.
- Psychological: euphoria, sensation of increased physical and mental well-being, these may be followed by irritability, depression and insomnia, paranoia may develop.

General/chronic
- Physical: runny nose, eczema localised around the nose, and nasal septum damage (erosions, necrosis, perforations) with anosmia can develop. Weight loss and malnutrition are common.
- Psychological: as for acute intoxication. Disturbance of eating and sleeping patterns may occur.

Cessation/withdrawal
Tolerance develops to the psychological effects but not the effects on the heart. Physical and psychological dependence occur and tend to be more severe if the drug is smoked or taken intravenously. The withdrawal syndrome or 'crash' results in depression, anxiety, irritability, insomnia and

COCAINE *continued*

increased risk of self-harm. Pronounced drowsiness may be apparent for many hours after cessation of use.

Treatment

• Intoxication: nil unless complications develop. Then supportive with monitoring of vital signs in hospital setting.

General/chronic
As for intoxication.

Withdrawal
Psychological support and counselling including treatment of depression and sleep disturbance.

ECSTASY AND RELATED METHYLATED AMPHETAMINES

Principal drugs

3,4 Methylenedioxymethamphetamine (MDMA),
3,4 methylenedioxyamphetamine (MDA) (see also Amphetamines).

Used in the dance/club culture for their central stimulant and psychedelic effects.

Manufacture
Laboratory/factory production.

Common street names
Ecstasy, 'E', doves, Dennis (the Menace), Adam (MDMA), Eve (MDA), sweet dreams, fantasy.

Mechanism of action
CNS stimulant with actions on the dopamine and serotonin pathways. Alteration in thermoregulation may occur due to action on the noradrenergic pathway.

Medical uses
Nil.

Legal status
Class A under Schedule 1 of the Misuse of Drugs Act 1971 (1977 Modification Order).

Presentation and methods of administration
Tablets (variable colours), capsules and powder, taken by mouth, snorted or smoked, rarely injected.

ECSTASY AND RELATED METHYLATED AMPHETAMINES *continued*

Symptoms and signs

Acute intoxication – similar to amphetamine and cocaine.
- Physical: effects take 20–60 min after ingestion and may last for several hours (4–6 h). These are dose-dependent – a moderate dose being between 75 and 100 mg: tachycardia, dry throat, jaw tightening, sweating, pyrexia, nausea and vomiting, transient anorexia, loss of co-ordination, headache, bruxism, trismus, nystagmus, blurring of vision, ataxia, muscle cramps, urinary urgency, brisk reflexes, paraesthesia.

In overdose or in susceptible individuals, convulsions, hyper- or hypotension, hyperthermia, cardiac dysrhythmias, disseminated intravascular coagulation (DIC), rhabdomyolysis and renal failure may occur. Deaths have been reported in association with the use of just one tablet (not caused by contaminants, as has been suggested). Some deaths have been related to cerebral oedema secondary to excess water ingestion, because the drug has an anti-diuretic effect on the kidney. The effects may be exacerbated or precipitated by associated physical activity.

- Psychological: a mild, euphoric 'rush', feelings of energy and vitality, increased self-esteem, increased self-confidence, visual and auditory hallucinations (rarely unpleasant), flashbacks may occur, anxiety attacks, aggression, insomnia, psychosis.

General/chronic
- Physical: as for acute intoxication. Physical dependence is not considered to occur, although tolerance does occur. Liver abnormalities have been reported.

Psychological
As for acute intoxication. Flashbacks may be increasingly experienced. Psychological dependence is not believed to occur. Depression, anxiety and memory disorders as well as psychotic illness may occur; there is some evidence that ecstasy causes damage to the serotonergic neurones in the brain.

Cessation/withdrawal
After the acute effects of the drug have worn off the user may experience several days of anxiety, depression and fatigue.

Treatment

- Intoxication: close observation of pulse rate, blood pressure, temperature and mental state. If any of these are abnormal observation should be within a hospital setting where facilities for supportive treatment (e.g. ventilation, intracranial pressure monitoring) and resuscitation are readily available.

GAMMAHYDROXYBUTYRATE

Principal drugs

Gammahydroxybutyrate (GHB).

Common street names
GHB, GBH, liquid E, liquid X, easylay, scoop salty water.

Mechanism of action
Anaesthetic with a sedative rather than analgesic effect. A naturally occurring substance structurally related to GABA and may be an inhibitory neurotransmitter. Effects occur between 10 min and an hour and dependent on dose may last for 24 h. Peak plasma levels within 20–40 min. Very short half-life rendering it difficult to detect, unless specifically suspected and searched for.

Medical uses
It has been used as a premedication.

Legal status
Not controlled under the Misuse of Drugs Act 1971, however GHB is classed as a medicine, so unauthorised manufacture and distribution could be an offence under the Medicines Act 1968.

Presentation and methods of administration
Colourless, odourless liquid may also be available in powder or capsules. Sold as a sodium salt – used on the street for bodybuilding, weight loss. Implicated in drug-facilitated sexual assault. Taken orally. May be used concurrently with other drugs (e.g. alcohol, cocaine, ecstasy). Rarely injected.

Symptoms and signs

Acute intoxication
- Physical: effects vary dependent on dose taken; lower doses (0–30 mg/kg) euphoria, agitation initially then sedation, nausea and

GAMMAHYDROXYBUTYRATE *continued*

vomiting, stiffening of muscles, disorientation; increasing doses (50 mg/kg) drowsiness, convulsions, coma, bradycardia, hypotension, Cheyne-Stokes respiration, respiratory collapse. There is a narrow margin between intoxication and coma and the effects are worse when mixed with other CNS depressants (e.g. alcohol and benzodiazepines). Recovery may be rapid – within a few hours. Although 'hang-over' and dizziness may persist for days.

Long-term effects
Unknown, but physical and psychological dependence may occur.

Treatment

There are no specific treatments – supportive care.

KETAMINE

Principal drugs

Ketamine.

Common street names
Special K, Vitamin K, Super K, Kit-Kat.

Mechanism of action
Dissociative anaesthetic and CNS depressant. Oral effects start within 20 min and can last up to 4 h, intravenous effects are experienced within minutes and usually last approximately 30 min.

Medical uses
Intravenous general anaesthetic agent with associated amnesia and analgesia. Used in veterinary medicine.

Legal status
POM under the Medicines Act, not controlled under the Misuse of Drugs Act 1971.

Presentation and methods of administration
Ketamine hydrochloride, found on the 'street' in capsules, crystals, powder or tablets. It can be taken orally, or smoked and snorted intranasally or injected via intramuscular or intravenous routes. Has been implicated in drug-facilitated sexual assault.

Symptoms and signs

Acute intoxication
- Physical: cocaine-like 'rush' – euphoria, agitation, aggression, vomiting and nausea, dysarthria, nystagmus, ataxia, loss of co-ordination, pronounced analgesia, cardio-respiratory stimulant in low doses, with an increase in blood pressure and pulse. High doses given rapidly intravenously may result in the depression of respiration or apnoea, which is especially dangerous with other CNS depressants. Rarely depression of the laryngeal reflexes predisposing to aspiration and airway obstruction may occur.
- Psychological: euphoria, psychological dissociation with hallucinations, stereotypia, synaesthesia. May experience 'out of body' effects.

In overdose or relative overdose – can experience fits, polyneuropathy, pulmonary oedema, respiratory failure, cardiac and respiratory arrest.

Chronic
Little information is available, but there may be interference with memory, learning and attention. The user may experience flashbacks. Tolerance can develop. There is generally no physical dependence or withdrawal although in those with ready access to supplies, dependence has been reported.

Treatment

After non-medical oral or nasal use all that may be required is rest in a quiet, darkened room. High doses: intensive observation may be required with mechanical support of respiration. Diazepam may have a role in some cases.

KHAT (QAT)

An alkaloid (cathinone) – derived from the leaves of the khat (qat) shrub – *Catha edulis*. Originates from Middle East and East Africa. Structurally similar to amphetamine (see Amphetamine).

Principal drugs and derivatives

Cathinone, cathine. Cathinone is broken down to cathine and noradrenaline. Cathine is excreted in urine, may be detected in urine within

KHAT (QAT) *continued*

50 min of ingestion – most is excreted by 24 h, peak plasma levels are 1–2 h after ingestion.

Manufacture
Cultivated.

Common street names
Khat, qat, catha, qaadka.

Mechanism of action
CNS stimulant.

Medical uses
None.

Legal status
Not illegal in plant form. May be bought in the UK as bundles of stalks and leaves. Cathine and cathinone are Class C drugs under Schedule 2 of the Misuse of Drugs Act 1971. Cathine is a Schedule 3 drug under the same Act. Thus once in liquid or tea form, it is illegal.

Presentation and methods of administration
Fresh leaves or stalks of the *Catha edulis* plant which are chewed. May be drunk as an infusion of leaves (Abyssinian Tea).

Symptoms and signs

Acute intoxication
- Physical: excitable and talkative, anorexia, tachycardia, insomnia, restlessness, dilated pupils, hypertension, palpitations, tremor, flushing. Impotence may be experienced. The mouth and tongue may become inflamed and painful (glossitis). Green-staining of the tongue may be noted if recent chewing has occurred. Gastritis may be present.
- Psychological: sense of well-being, irritability, euphoria, excitable, agitated, hyperactivity, hypo/hypermania.

General/chronic
There appears to be little physical dependence but psychological dependence occurs. Long-term use may cause bruxism, personality change. Psychosis (with visual and auditory hallucinations), although rare has been reported in predisposed individuals. Paranoid delusions may occur. There may be an increased incidence of peptic ulceration.

KHAT (QAT) *continued*

Cessation/withdrawal
Long-term users may experience tremor, lassitude and depression on withdrawal.

Treatment

- Intoxication: no specific treatment necessary.
- General/chronic: no specific treatment required.
- Withdrawal: if withdrawal effects are observed psychological support and counselling may be required.

LSD

Principal drugs and derivatives

An hallucinogen. A semi-synthetic drug derived from the alkaloid lysergic acid. D-lysergic acid diethylamide or lysergide or LSD-25. Lysergic acid is found in ergot, a fungus, which grows on grains such as rye. LSD was first synthesised from lysergic acid in 1938 in Switzerland.

Manufacture
Laboratory/factory production.

Common street names
Acid, tabs, dots, the cube, microdots, pellets, blue star, trips, California sunshine (and also by the names of the designs used in the manufacture of impregnated paper squares – e.g. Smiley, Gorby's, Oms, Strawberries).

Mechanism of action
Following oral intake, effects are evident within 60 min. The effects last up to 12 h, peaking at about 4 h. It acts on both central and autonomic nervous systems. It is metabolised in the liver and kidneys, with faecal excretion.

Medical uses
None. In its earlier years attempts were made to find a use, particularly in psychiatric disorder.

Legal status
Class A controlled drug under Schedule 2 of the Misuse of Drugs Act 1971.

LSD *continued*

Presentation and methods of administration
The amount of LSD required for an effect is minute (between 25–150 μg is adequate). It may be produced in the form of tablets, or impregnated on to paper, sugar cubes or gelatin squares.

Symptoms and signs

Acute intoxication
- Physical: increased blood pressure, pyrexia, headache, dilatation of the pupils, tachycardia. Tremor, flushing, nausea and temporary loss of appetite may be noted. Some temporary muscular inco-ordination may be experienced.
- Psychological: LSD is known as one of the most potent 'mind-expanding' drugs. Both enjoyable and unpleasant effects (a 'bad trip') may be experienced by users. Its effects vary greatly from individual to individual and vary in effect in each individual on repeated use. The effects vary with the individual's current state of mind, their personality and their environment. Visual hallucinations associated with visual distortion may be experienced. Auditory hallucinations are less common. Perception of time may alter, sometimes passing very slowly, and sometimes extremely quickly. The ability to judge distance or speed is reduced. Mood may change acutely from extreme happiness to the depths of depression. Paranoia may be felt, and episodes of violence have been described. As the effects of the drug wear off (over a few hours) periods of normality gradually return. In overdose or relative overdose – can experience fits, polyneuropathy, pulmonary oedema, respiratory failure, cardiac and respiratory arrest.

General/chronic
Psychological and physical dependence do not occur as tolerance develops rapidly.

- Psychological: prolonged psychotic and anxiety reactions occasionally occur. Flashbacks may occur weeks or months following use.

Cessation/withdrawal
Withdrawal is not considered a problem, as the nature of the drug generally prevents regular (e.g. daily) use.

Treatment

- Intoxication: supportive treatment whilst 'trip' is underway.

LSD *continued*

- General/chronic: no specific treatment is required. Disturbing flashbacks have been treated with benzodiazepines.
- Withdrawal: no specific treatment is required.

NITRITES

Principal drugs

Amyl nitrite, butyl nitrite, sodium nitrite, isobutyl nitrite, sildenafil.

Common street names
Poppers, TNT, rock hard, rush.

Mechanism of action
All the nitrites dilate blood vessels by relaxing the muscles in the walls of the vessels. Inhalation of the vapour results in an almost instantaneous but short-lived effect. Use of 'poppers' in combination with sildenafil (Viagra™) may result in fainting due to the combined effect of lowering the blood pressure.

Medical uses
Sodium nitrite is used as an antidote to cyanide poisoning.

Legal status
Amyl nitrite is classified under the Medicines Act as a pharmacy only medicine, butyl nitrite is not classified as a drug and therefore there are no restrictions on its availability. Sildenafil is a POM prescribed for erectile dysfunction.

Presentation and methods of administration
A clear yellow volatile inflammable liquid with a sweet smell. It is manufactured in a small glass capsule but as street drugs is usually found in a bottle. The substance can be inhaled directly from the bottle or poured onto a cloth. They are also popular amongst young people as an euphoric relaxant within dance culture. Sildenafil is produced as a blue tablet.

Symptoms and signs

Acute intoxication
- Physical: euphoria, tachycardia, hypotension, headache, dizziness, light-headedness, flushed face, weakness and nausea.

At higher doses nausea and vomiting, weakness, fainting, bradycardia.

NITRITES *continued*

Chronic
• Facial dermatitis, allergic rash and anaemia. Methaemoglobinaemia may occur. Tolerance does occur after a couple of weeks of regular use. There is no evidence of a physical or psychological dependence.

Treatment

There are no specific treatments.

OPIOIDS

Principal drugs

Diamorphine or heroin, morphine, dipipanone, methadone, pethidine, dextromoramide, dextropropoxyphene, pentazocine, buprenorphine, codeine.

Common street names
Brown, Chinese, Skag, smack, H, dike, amps, Harry, gear, linctus, elephant, tackle, crap, shit, gear (these predominantly refer to heroin).

Mechanism of action
Opiates are narcotic drugs and analgesics that depress the CNS through suppression of noradrenaline; when abstinence occurs there is a rebound release of noradrenaline causing withdrawal.

Medical uses
Include pain relief, cough suppressant, anti-diarrhoea agents and treatment of opiate dependence (methadone and buprenorphine).

Legal status
POM and are controlled under the Misuse of Drugs Act 1971 making it illegal to possess them without a prescription. Morphine, opium, methadone, dipipanone and pethidine are in Class A of the Act, dihydrocodeine and codeine in Class B and dextropropoxyphene and buprenorphine Class C (see Drugs, Statutes and Legal Requirements).

Presentation and methods of administration
Tablets, linctus, injectable liquid if manufactured, a white powder if illicit. Heroin can be smoked, sniffed or injected (as 'brown', heroin will need to be dissolved in an acid – usually citric acid – before intravenous injection), most other preparations can be injected or taken orally. Intravenous injection

(mainlining) results in an almost instantaneous effect 'rush' whereas injection into muscle or subcutaneous injection (skin popping) gives a slower and less intense effect. Sniffing will also result in a less intense effect but the effects of smoking ('chasing the dragon') are almost as quick as intravenous injection.

Preparations include:

Methadone, a synthetic opiate analgesic with onset of action of 30 min and a long duration of action of 24–36 h. It is available in various preparations including: physeptone tablets containing methadone hydrochloride 5 mg; methadone mixture (see below); methadone injection clear colourless ampoules of 1 ml, 2 ml, 3.5 ml and 5 ml containing a colourless solution of methadone hydrochloride BP 10 mg per ml.

Diconal contains dipipanone with the anti-histamine cyclizine which is effective in preventing the nausea and vomiting associated with narcotic analgesics. It appears that cyclizine enhances the effects of opiates and is commonly taken by injection.

Buprenorphine is a partial agonist with a long duration of action. It is an effective analgesic and can be taken sublingually or by injection. After chronic administration the onset of the withdrawal syndrome is delayed with only mild signs from 3–10 days. The tablets are sometimes crushed and injected.

Symptoms and signs

Acute intoxication
- Physical: pinpoint (constricted) pupils, depression of the heart rate and respiration, suppression of the cough reflex, constipation, drowsiness and sleep. Nausea and vomiting can occur. High doses can result in respiratory arrest, unconsciousness and death. There may be fatal reactions to the impurities injected with illicit heroin.
- Psychological: opioids reduce anxiety, produce pain relief and euphoria, a feeling of contentment, inability to concentrate and memory difficulties. The general depressant effects of methadone may be enhanced by other agents with CNS depressant activity such as alcohol, barbiturates, tricyclic anti-depressants and phenothiazines. The analgesic effects of opioid drugs tend to be enhanced by the co-administration of dexamphetamine.

Chronic
Tolerance and physical and psychological dependence occur. However, tolerance does not develop to all the effects of opiates as increasing doses

OPIOIDS *continued*

have to be taken to achieve the same analgesic or euphoric effect but pupillary constriction will usually remain constant. Cross-tolerance does occur between the various opiates. If drug administration is stopped, for example by a period of imprisonment, then tolerance will be lost and there is a risk that if the previous dose is taken fatal intoxication will occur. The severity of physical dependence depends on the particular opiate used, the dose and the duration of administration. Psychological dependence on opiates is severe and persists after the physical withdrawal syndrome has passed. There is therefore a high relapse rate of opiate addiction. Amenorrhoea and loss of libido occur and chronic constipation. Women generally remain fertile despite the menstrual irregularity. Opiate use during pregnancy may result in 'small for dates' babies who themselves may suffer severe withdrawal symptoms after birth.

Withdrawal

The onset, peak and duration of symptoms of the withdrawal syndrome will depend on which opiate is misused, for example heroin withdrawal will have an earlier onset (within 8 h progress to a peak and then improve slowly over 48–72 h), will be of shorter duration and of greater intensity as compared with methadone (2–6 days and 10–12 days respectively). The expectation of withdrawal and psychological factors are also important.

- Symptoms: yawning, feelings of hot and cold, anorexia, abdominal cramps, nausea, vomiting, diarrhoea, tremor, insomnia, restlessness, generalised aches and pains, weakness.
- Signs: dilated pupils, gooseflesh, flushing, sweating, rhinorrhoea or lachrymation, tachycardia (a pulse rate of 10 beats per minute over the baseline or over 90 beats per minute if no history of tachycardia), hypertension (systolic blood pressure 10 mmHg or more above baseline or over 160/96 in non-hypertensive patients), increased bowel sounds.

Opiate withdrawal during pregnancy can result in fetal death and premature labour. Therefore maintenance therapy with substitute opioids is preferred.

Treatment

- Overdose: naloxone is a specific opioid antagonist and is given in a dose of 0.4 mg which can be repeated at intervals of 2–3 min up to a maximum of 10 mg. If there is no effect then the diagnosis of opiate overdose should be reconsidered. Naloxone has a short half-life and therefore observation in hospital is required after treatment. Naloxone can be given intravenously or intramuscularly (it may be difficult to establish intravenous access) where it has a longer duration of action.

Naloxone administration is not without risk in the opiate dependent individual and it may precipitate the opiate withdrawal syndrome which is distressing but short-lived. Rarely hypertension, pulmonary oedema and cardiac dysrhythmias may occur.

Naltrexone is also a specific opioid antagonist in tablet form and is used as an adjunctive therapy in the maintenance of detoxified formerly opioid dependent patients.

Withdrawal

The following drugs can be used in the symptomatic treatment of opiate withdrawal:

- Benzodiazepines, nitrazepam or chlordiazepoxide can be used to relieve anxiety and insomnia.
- Diphenoxylate and atropine (Lomotil™), two tablets four times a day or loperamide (Imodium™) 2 mg four times daily for diarrhoea and gut spasm.
- Promethazine, an anti-emetic with sedative properties in a dose of 10–20 mg three times a day or 25 mg at night.
- Paracetamol, and other non-steroidal anti-inflammatory drugs are useful for minor aches and pains.
- Buscopan, 10 mg four times a day for gut spasm.
- Clonidine, is an alpha-adrenergic drug which should be used in the hospital setting as it causes sedation and hypotension. It is not licenced but it is useful in certain cases.
- Lofexidine, is a structural analogue of clonidine but it is less sedating and less hypotensive (dose 0.2–0.4 mg four times a day for 4 days).
- Buprenorphine (Subutex™) is licenced as an adjunct in the treatment of opioid dependence and has been used widely in some countries.
- Substitution – Methadone, codeine or dihydrocodeine can be used (see Table 6).

OPIOIDS *continued*

Table 6 Opiate equivalents for treatment of withdrawal

	Drug	Dose
1 mg of methadone mixture* is equivalent to:	Buprenorphine	20 µg
	Codeine	30 mg
	Dextromoramide	2 mg
	Dextropropoxyphene	20 mg
	Dihydrocodeine	10 mg
	Dipinanone	2 mg
	Methadone linctus	1 mg/2.5 ml
	Methadone Mixture	1 mg/ml
	Morphine	3.4 mg
	Pethidine	20 mg
	Pharmaceutical heroin	20 µg

*Care must be taken when administering, prescribing or taking a history as methadone is available in a number of strengths and colours (methadone mixture 1 mg/ml – green colour; oral concentrate 10 mg/ml – blue and 20 mg/ml – brown).

As a general rule the starting dose should not exceed 40 mg of methadone mixture or equivalent.

If there is doubt regarding the daily dose of methadone this can be divided and the condition of the patient reviewed after a proportion has been administered. Naltrexone is a pure opiate antagonist with a long half-life. It can be taken orally and blocks the effects of opiates for 72 h therefore it can be administered three times a week. It should not be given to an individual who is still dependent on opiates until 7–10 days after the last ingestion of opiates otherwise it will precipitate a withdrawal reaction which will be protracted because of the long duration of action of naltrexone.

PCP

Principal drugs and derivatives

Dissociative anaesthetic and hallucinogen. Phencyclidine or phencyclidine hydrochloride or 1-[1-phenylcyclohexyl] piperidine.

Manufacture
Laboratory/factory production.

PCP *continued*

Common street names
Angel dust, dust, crystal, rocket fuel.

Mechanism of action
Dependent on dosage may act as an anaesthetic, a stimulant, a depressant or as an hallucinogen. It has mixed neurological effects.

PCP is absorbed rapidly after smoking or injection with effects within minutes (5–15); orally peak effects after 2 h. Acute effects will last for 4–6 h, with a return to normality within 24 h. PCP may be detected in blood and urine for up to one week.

Medical uses
Originally used as a human anaesthetic agent but later limited to veterinary medicine. No current medical use.

Legal status
Class A drug under Schedule 2 of the Misuse of Drugs Act 1971.

Presentation and methods of administration
A crystalline white powder, readily soluble in water or alcohol. May be smoked, taken orally, intranasally or injected usually intravenously.

Symptoms and signs

There is wide variation among users dependent on dose and the setting in which the drug is taken, the user's expectation, past drug experience and personality.

Acute intoxication
- Physical: loss of co-ordination, slurred speech, sweating, tachycardia, tachypnoea and hypertension. Nystagmus, visual disturbance and nausea may be experienced. The anaesthetic properties of PCP may render the individual less sensitive to pain, allowing injuries to go unnoticed. Death due to convulsions, respiratory arrest and hypertension have been reported.
- Psychological: euphoria, relaxation, drowsiness, feelings of dissociation, perceptual disturbances, visual and auditory distortions.

General/chronic
- Physical: no physical dependence is thought to occur.
- Psychological: there is some evidence that psychological dependence develops. Memory may be affected. Drug-induced psychosis following use of PCP may last up to several weeks, particularly in those with

PCP *continued*

a history of psychiatric disorder such as schizophrenia. Tolerance may develop. Craving for the drug may occur.

Cessation/withdrawal
Depression and social withdrawal are common sequelae of chronic PCP misuse. There may be a mild abstinence syndrome with depression and disorientation.

Treatment

- Intoxication – acidification of the urine may reduce the drug half-life by accelerating excretion.
- General/chronic – no specific treatment.
- Withdrawal – standard treatment(s) for depressive episodes when clinically indicated.

TOBACCO

Tobacco is produced from the tobacco plant – *Nicotiana tabacum*.

Principal drugs and derivatives

The content of tobacco smoke is complex, about 500 different compounds have been identified. The predominant pharmacologically active ingredients are nicotine and tars. Nicotine is an oily alkaloid. Pure nicotine is extremely poisonous – a dose of 50 mg can cause death within minutes.

Manufacture
Tobacco plants are commercially cultivated and harvested worldwide.

Common street names
Ciggies, tabs, roll-ups, fags.

Mechanism of action
Nicotine is both stimulant and sedative with effects on the CNS and the voluntary and involuntary nervous systems – this is dose-dependent. In the doses used in smoking nicotine causes release of catecholamines, serotonin, anti-diuretic hormone, corticotrophin and growth hormone. Nicotine inhaled as smoke will reach the brain within 1 min. Its effects on the body last for about 30 min. It is excreted in urine following metabolism to inert substances.

Medical uses
None.

Legal status
Tobacco products may not be bought by those under 16 years of age.

Presentation and methods of administration
Dried leaves of the tobacco plant may be smoked in cigarettes (manufactured or 'roll-ups'), cigars and pipes. Leaves may be chewed. Ground up dried tobacco may be taken as snuff. One cigarette may contain up to 20 mg of nicotine – lower nicotine brands may be as low as 0.5 mg. A cigarette may contain up to 15 mg tars, low-tar brands containing considerably less.

Symptoms and signs

Acute intoxication
- Physical: tachycardia, hypertension, sore throat, sore eyes, tremor.
- Psychological: some individuals feel more alert, some feel more tranquil.

General/chronic
- Physical: dependence develops rapidly (within days). Long-term smoking is associated with a large range of diseases and illnesses including, lung cancer, atherosclerosis (manifest as angina, myocardial infarction, cerebrovascular accidents, peripheral vascular disease), bronchitis, peptic ulcers, reduced fertility (females), complications of pregnancy (including smaller babies), cancers of the mouth and throat. Children of female smokers may be shorter and have delayed intellectual development. All these risks increase the longer the individual has smoked. The risks vary according to the type of use (e.g. cigarettes v pipes) and the method of use (e.g. inhaling v not inhaling). Stopping smoking will eventually decrease the risk.
- Psychological: dependence is marked.

Cessation/withdrawal
A withdrawal syndrome develops with the individual experiencing fatigue, shortness of breath, headache and in the long-term, irritability and depression. This may last for several weeks after cessation. Many individuals become preoccupied with the absence of smoking. Weight gain may be observed because of a reduction in metabolic rate and 'comfort' eating.

TOBACCO *continued*

Treatment

- Intoxication: no specific treatment.
- General/chronic – the ease (or not) of stopping smoking varies with each individual. Some individuals may stop without support. The majority require assistance. Tapered nicotine replacement therapy (using nicotine-supplying gum or skin-patches) may be useful. Anxiolytic drugs, counselling, hypnotherapy, acupuncture all have their place in the management of those experiencing difficulties. Amfebutamone/bupropion is increasingly used as an adjunctive agent in smoking cessation.
- Withdrawal: no specific treatment.

VOLATILE SUBSTANCES

Principal drugs

Toluene, acetone, butane, fluorocarbons, trichloroethylene, trichloroethane.

Presentation and methods of administration
A variety of substances can be misused, for example solvents in adhesives (glue) such as toluene (the most commonly sniffed solvent), acetone in nail polish, fuel gases such as butane and propane, petrol, fluorocarbons in aerosols, cleaning agents such as trichloroethylene and trichloroethane, fire-extinguishing agents such as bromochlorodifluoromethane, benign aerosol propellants such as halon, the propellants in some inhalers and anaesthetic agents such as nitrous oxide or halothane.

Volatile substance abuse (VSA) is the inhalation of such fumes in order to achieve intoxication. Vapours or gases are inhaled through the nose or mouth with the method depending on the substance misused, for example some products can be sniffed directly from their containers; put in a plastic bag for inhalation – 'huffing'; poured onto clothing; be sprayed directly into the mouth.

Medical uses
Apart from the anaesthetic agents there are no recommended medical uses for these substances.

Mechanism of action
The solvents are rapidly absorbed through the lungs and pass rapidly into the blood stream. They are highly lipid soluble resulting in effects within minutes which wear off quickly although repeated doses may be taken.

VOLATILE SUBSTANCES *continued*

Legal status
Widely available in shops. The anaesthetic agents are POM under the Medicines Act. Under the Intoxicating Supply Act 1985 (England and Wales) it is illegal to sell volatile substances knowingly for inhalation. The Solvent Abuse Act 1983 (Scotland) made VSA one of the grounds for referring a young person to a Children's Panel.

Symptoms and signs

Acute intoxication — similar to alcohol intoxication usually with a more rapid onset.

- Physical: the solvent smell may be apparent on the breath, hands and clothing, nasal sores, burns, adhesive marks, 'glue-sniffer's rash' — perioral eczema, singed scalp hair, moustache, beard. Nausea, vomiting, diarrhoea, sneezing and coughing may occur. Giddiness, tachycardia, conjunctival injection, impaired judgement, sedation, nystagmus, poor co-ordination, slurred speech and ataxic gait.

High doses may result in depression of the CNS with seizures, coma and death.

Sudden death is a recognised complication of solvent misuse and may occur during exposure, in the post-exposure period or result from trauma or asphyxia secondary to intoxication. Death may result from anoxia, respiratory depression, vagal inhibition and cardiac dysrhythmias. Dysrhythmias may be difficult to treat and the risk remains for several hours after inhalation.

After the acute effects wear off there may be a 'hang-over' with drowsiness and headaches with poor concentration which may persist for up to a day.

- Psychological: euphoria with excitatory effects secondary to disinhibition (similar to alcohol but the effects occur more quickly). With increasing dosage there may be perceptual disturbances, hallucinations and delusions.

Chronic
- May result in fatigue, memory impairment with poor concentration.

Tolerance and psychological dependence may develop.

Very long-term misuse may result in a multitude of symptoms with resulting liver, heart or renal damage and nervous system involvement including cerebellar disease, dementia and peripheral neuropathy. Perioral eczema and upper respiratory tract problems may occur with chronic misuse.

VOLATILE SUBSTANCES *continued*

Treatment

• There are no specific treatments. Many effects are reversible on cessation of solvent misuse except when the product is highly toxic as with leaded petrol where brain damage has occurred through lead poisoning.

MISCELLANEOUS DRUGS

A number of hallucinogenic drugs are derived from readily available plants. The two most common, mescaline and psilocybin have effects similar to those of LSD. Although occurring naturally they may also be synthesised.

Mescaline was first used by Aztec Indians in Mexico and is derived from peyotl (Mexican cactus – *Lophorphora williamsii*). Its chemical structure was determined in 1918. The effects appear within 3–4 h of ingestion, and last up to 12. It is normally eaten, occasionally smoked and rarely injected. It does not cause serious dependence and is still used in certain religious ceremonies in the American continent. It is rarely seen in the UK.

'Magic Mushrooms' or 'Mushies' describes a group of wild mushrooms which may cause hallucinations and visual disturbance. The active drug is psilocybin. Psilocybin is derived from the several varieties of Psilocybe mushrooms. In the UK the most common is *Psilocybe semilanceata* – the Liberty Cap. Psilocybin was isolated in 1958. It is normally eaten – as 'Magic Mushrooms' – and rarely injected. It is rapid-acting the effects being observed within 15 min of ingestion, lasting up to about 6 h.

Possession of 'Magic Mushrooms' is not illegal, unless they have been prepared for illicit use. Mescaline, psilocybin and psilocyn are Class A drugs under Schedule 2 to the Misuse of Drugs Act 1971.

GLOSSARY OF MEDICAL AND 'STREET' DRUG-RELATED TERMS

The street terms for drugs expands and changes with regularity – as with those terms mentioned in relation to specific drugs, the terms below are those accepted medically, or have had regular street usage.

Abstinence – the act of refraining from the use of a substance which may lead to withdrawal syndromes such as delirium tremens or barbiturate withdrawal.

Anosmia – loss of sense of smell.

Ataxia – disturbance of co-ordination of movement.

Bruxism – grinding of teeth.

CNS – central nervous system.

Detoxification – is the process whereby drug withdrawal is managed in a person dependent on alcohol or other drugs.

Drug – any substance, other than those required for the maintenance of normal health, that, when taken into the living organism may modify one or more of its functions (World Health Organisation).

DIC – disseminated intravascular coagulation.

Drug dependence (also chemical or substance dependence) – a state, psychic and sometimes also physical, resulting from the interaction between a living organism and a drug, characterised by behavioural and other responses that always include a compulsion to take the drug on a continuous or periodic basis in order to experience its psychic effects and sometimes to avoid discomfort of its absence (World Health Organisation).

Drug misuse – has been defined as any taking of a drug which harms or threatens to harm the physical and mental health or social well-being of an individual, or of other individuals, or of society at large, or which is illegal (Royal College of Psychiatrists 1987).

Drug paraphernalia – items associated with drug use, e.g. syringes, needles, foil, citric acid, scales.

Dysarthria – slurred speech – difficulty in articulation.

Dysrhythmia (*cardiac*) – irregularity of heartbeat.

Flashbacks – spontaneous involuntary recurrences of drug-induced experiences.

IVDU – intravenous drug user.

Maintenance treatment – continued use of substitution treatment as an alternative to detoxification and may be required where an individual has relapsed on several occasions after detoxification.

Nystagmus – spontaneous rapid rhythmic eye movements in a side-to-side (horizontal) or up-and-down (vertical) direction.

Oedema – swelling.

Paraesthesia – altered sensation.

Polydrug misuse – occurs when a person misuses more than one drug. For example it is not uncommon to find an individual addicted to opiates and benzodiazepines.

POM – prescription only medicine.

Recreational use (of a drug) – the use of a drug intermittently for pleasure, not associated with dependence to that drug.

Rehabilitation – restoration of normal function.

Rush – an immediate sensation of well-being after taking a substance.

Skin pop – the practice of injecting drugs into tissue under the skin, often leaving circular depressed scars.

Stereotypia – persistent repetition of words or movements.

Synaesthesia – the experience of 'hearing colours' and 'seeing sounds'.

Tolerance (to a drug) – the need to increase the drug dose to get the same effect or where the same dose of a drug produces a reduced effect – occurs after repeated use of certain drugs as the body adapts.

Tracks – the line(s) (often discoloured like a bruise) along a vein where impure materials (most injectable illicit drugs) have been injected. May be evident for many days or weeks or even longer.

Trismus – clenching of teeth.

VSA – volatile substance abuse.

Withdrawal – the individual or cluster of symptoms and signs which are associated with the abstinence from long-term use of some drugs (e.g. delirium tremens).

Works – needles and syringes used for injection.

BIBLIOGRAPHY

Association of Police Surgeons and Royal College of Psychiatrists. Substance misuse detainees in police custody – guidelines for clinical management. Report of a Medical Working Group, June 2000.

Drummer OH. The Forensic Pharmacology of Drugs of Abuse. Arnold, London, 2001.

Fortson R. Misuse of Drugs and Drug Trafficking Offences 4th ed. Sweet and Maxwell, London.

Department of Health. Drug Misuse and Dependence – Guidelines on Clinical Management. The Stationery Office, London, 1999.

Jones AL, Dargan PI. Pocketbook of Toxicology. Churchill Livingstone, Edinburgh 2001.

Karch SB. Karch's Pathology of Drug Abuse 3rd ed. CRC Press LLC, Boca Raton, 2002.

Payne-James JJ, Busuttil A, Smock WS. Forensic Medicine: Clinical and Pathological Aspects. Greenwich Medical Media; London, 2003.

Stark MM. A Physician's Guide to Clinical Forensic Medicine. Humana Press, Totowa, New Jersey, 2000.

CONVERSION CHART FOR HEIGHT

ft	in	m	ft	in	m
4	0	1.22	5	8	1.73
4	1	1.25	5	9	1.75
4	2	1.27	5	10	1.78
4	3	1.30	5	11	1.80
4	4	1.32	6	0	1.83
4	5	1.35	6	1	1.85
4	6	1.37	6	2	1.88
4	7	1.40	6	3	1.90
4	8	1.42	6	4	1.93
4	9	1.45	6	5	1.96
4	10	1.47	6	6	1.98
4	11	1.50	6	7	2.01
5	0	1.52	6	8	2.03
5	1	1.55	6	9	2.06
5	2	1.58	6	10	2.08
5	3	1.60	6	11	2.11
5	4	1.63	7	0	2.13

Extracts from the BSI Height and Weight Conversion Chart are reproduced with permission. Copies of the chart can be obtained by post from BSI Sales, Linford Wood, Milton Keynes, UK.

CONVERSION CHART FOR WEIGHT

st	lb	kg	st	lb	kg	st	lb	kg
5	0	31.6	10	6	66.2	15	12	100.7
5	2	32.7	10	8	67.1	16	0	101.6
5	4	33.6	10	10	68.0	16	3	102.9
5	6	34.5	10	12	68.9	16	6	104.3
5	8	35.4	11	0	68.9	16	9	105.7
5	10	36.3	11	2	70.7	16	12	107.0
5	12	37.2	11	4	71.7	17	0	107.9
6	0	38.1	11	6	72.7	17	3	109.3
6	2	30.0	11	8	73.5	17	6	110.7
6	4	39.9	11	10	74.4	17	9	112.0
6	6	40.8	11	12	75.3	17	12	113.4
6	8	41.7	12	0	76.2	18	0	114.3
6	10	42.6	12	2	77.1	18	3	115.7
6	12	43.5	12	4	78.0	18	6	117.0
7	0	44.5	12	6	78.9	18	9	118.4
7	2	45.4	12	8	79.8	18	12	119.7
7	4	46.3	12	10	80.7	19	0	120.7
7	6	47.2	12	12	81.6	19	3	122.0
7	8	48.1	13	0	82.6	19	6	123.3
7	10	48.9	13	2	83.5	19	9	124.7
7	12	49.9	13	4	84.4	19	12	126.1
8	0	50.8	13	6	85.3	20	0	127.0

Extract from the BSI Height and Weight Conversion Chart are reproduced with permission. Copies of the chart can be obtained by post from BSI Sales, Linford Wood, Milton Keynes, UK.

GLASGOW COMA SCORE

Category	Score
Best performance	
Eye opening	
spontaneous	4
to speech	3
to pain	2
nil	1
Verbal response	
oriented	5
confused	4
inappropriate	3
incomprehensible	2
nil	1
Motor response	
obeying commands	5
localising	4
flexing	3
extending	2
nil	1

FIELD IMPAIRMENT TESTING PROCESS
(Section 4 – Road Traffic Act, 1988)

ADDITIONAL WARNING – to be given in all cases

I would like you to perform a series of tests to enable me to ascertain whether there are grounds to suspect that your ability to drive is impaired by drink or drugs. **(I must tell you that you are not under arrest and you need not remain with me.) You are not obliged to participate in the tests but if you do participate, the results may be given in evidence. The tests are simple and part of my evaluation will be based on your ability to follow instructions. If you do not understand any of the instructions, please tell me so that I may clarify them. ** Not to be read if the person has already been arrested <u>Do you understand?</u>

<u>Do you agree to participate in these tests?</u>

As I explain the test to you, if you have any medical condition or disability which may affect your ability to undertake the tests or it's results, please tell me before the test is started. <u>Do you understand?</u>

<u>Do you have any medical condition or disability that you wish to tell me about before I start the test?</u>

---

1. PUPILLARY EXAMINATION

I am going to examine the size of your pupils, comparing them to this gauge, which I shall hold up to the side of your face. All I require you to do is look straight ahead and keep your eyes open. **DO YOU UNDERSTAND?**

2. ROMBERG TEST

Stand up straight with your feet together and your arms by your side. Maintain that position whilst I give you the remaining instructions. Do not begin until I tell you to start. When I tell you to start, you must tilt your head back slightly and close your eyes (*Demonstrate but do not close eyes*). Keep your head tilted backwards with your eyes closed until you think that 30 seconds has passed, then bring your head forward and say 'Stop'. **DO YOU UNDERSTAND?**

At the end ask "HOW LONG WAS THAT?"

3. WALK AND TURN

(Find a real or imaginary line. Do not use a kerb or anywhere the subject may fall). Place your left foot on the line. Place your right foot on the line in front of the left foot touching heel to toe **(Demonstrate)**. Put your arms by your sides and keep them there throughout the entire test. Maintain that position while I give you the remaining instructions. **DO YOU UNDERSTAND?** When I say start, you must take nine heel to toe steps along the line. On each step the heel of the foot must be placed against the toe of the other foot **(Demonstrate)**. When the ninth step has been taken, you must leave the front foot on the line and turn around using a series of small steps with the other foot. After turning you must take another nine heel to toe steps along the line. You must watch your feet at all times and count each step out loud. Once you start walking do not stop until you have completed the test. **DO YOU UNDERSTAND?** *(Demonstrate complete test)*

4. ONE LEG STAND

Stand with your feet together and your arms down by your sides. Maintain that position while I give you the remaining instructions. Do not begin until I tell you to start. **DO YOU UNDERSTAND?** When I tell you to start, you must raise your right foot 6 to 8 inches off the ground, keeping your leg straight and your toes pointing forward, with your foot parallel to the ground. **(Demonstrate)**. You must keep your arms down by your sides and keep looking at your elevated foot while counting out loud in the following manner, One thousand and one, One thousand and two and so on until I tell you to stop. **DO YOU UNDERSTAND?** *(Repeat with other foot)*

5. FINGER TO NOSE

Stand with your feet together and your arms in this position. *(Demonstrate extending both hands out in front, palms side up and closed with the index finger of both hands extended)*. Maintain that position while I give you the remaining instructions. Do not begin until I tell you to start. When I tell you to start you must tilt your head slightly backwards and close your eyes. When I tell you which hand to move, you must touch the tip of your nose with the tip of that finger and lower your hand once you have done so **(Demonstrate) DO YOU UNDERSTAND?** *(Call out hands in following order, Left, Right, Left, Right, Right, Left.)*

Acknowledgement: Reproduced with kind permission of Home Office.

1.0
1.5
2.0
2.5
3.0
3.5
4.0
4.5
5.0
5.5
6.0
6.5
7.0
7.5
8.0
8.5
9.0

INDEX